ALLERGIES

A NUTRITIONAL APPROACH

by Louise Tenney, M.H.

© 1996

Woodland Publishing Inc.
P.O. Box 160
Pleasant Grove, UT 84062

TABLE OF CONTENTS

What are allergies and why are they triggered? This question as puzzled the scientific community for years. While all the whys nd wherefores of allergies remain somewhat of a mystery, hrough continuing research, the pieces of the puzzle are finally oming together.

There are few things that can cause the misery of allergy ymptoms which affect large segments of the world's population. or allergy victims, green grasses, blossoms, and leafy trees can ctivate miserable sneezing attacks, itchy, watery eyes and swollen inuses. While these are typical allergy symptoms, more subtle nanifestations can occur with food allergies, and of course, in the ase of some allergies to bee stings, nuts or penicillin, an allergy an be life-threatening.

WHAT IS AN ALLERGY

The T-cells of our immune system act to safeguard our bodies gainst foreign invaders. When a foreign substance enters our ellular systems, these T-cells spring into action and attempt to radicate the invader through a series of physiological responses. echnically, an allergy is a disorder which occurs when our lefense system overreacts to the presence of benign substances erceived as potentially harmful. It is technically a malfunction of ur immune system, which attacks substances such as dust or ollen with sticky proteins called antibodies. Several of these ubstances, which can be eaten, inhaled or come into contact with he surface of the skin can cause an allergic reaction in certain ndividuals.When the immune system is stimulated by the resence of an allergen, antibodies produce histamine and erotonin, which cause inflammation resulting in itching, neezing, runny nose etc.

These intolerances can trigger severe reactions and symptoms vhich manifest themselves in a variety of ways. Recent clinical tudies have concluded that allergic reactions can extend beyond ust red eyes and sniffles. Allergies have been implicated in yperactivity, mental illnesses, arthritis, and a whole host of other eemingly unrelated ailments.

CAUSES OF ALLERGIES

Allergic reactions can be caused by certain foods, pollens, danders, dust mites and insect venoms. In addition, certain met (particularly nickel), lanolin, some cosmetic ingredients, cert drugs such as penicillin and aspirin, food additives, preservativ and foods such as milk, eggs, strawberries, wheat, nuts a shellfish are all notorious for their connection to allergies. Infar and young children can be sensitive to cow's milk which c cause skin rashes, colic and diarrhea.

While the exact reason why a certain individual becom allergic to the substances mentioned above remains unclear a somewhat controversial, heredity is a major determining fact Additionally, some health experts believe that babies who are n breast fed are more likely to develop certain allergies. Introduci foods such as citrus fruits, cow's milk or wheat prematurely in an infant's diet have also been linked to allergies.

The pollens which come from ragweed and other plants ca also cause seasonal allergies. Certain varieties of grasses a considered allergens for thousands of people. In addition, conta with dog, cat or horse dander frequently trigger an allerg response. Mold and house dust are both allergic culprits as well insect bites and stings. Drug sensitivities to penicillin which made from a mold can cause severe allergic reactions.

Significant links between emotional stress and the onset of a allergy have also been observed. Stress and anger have bee known to bring on allergic symptoms, especially if the immur system has been compromised.

SYMPTOMS OF AN ALLERGY

The intensity of an allergic reaction can range from simple ha fever, hives and asthma to potentially fatal anaphylactic shock. It important to remember that the term "allergy" is frequentl misused. Skin irritations which are the result of contact wit certain chemicals, and coughing caused from exposure to cigaret smoke are not necessarily the result of a true, allergic reaction.

It is very difficult to completely list all of the causes an symptoms of allergies. Practically anything is capable c roducing an allergic response. In addition, autoimmune diseases nvolve a complex allergic reaction to one's own body fluids.

.llergies can include one or a combination of the following ymptoms:

- HIVES
- ITCHY SWOLLEN PALMS
- SKIN RASHES
- SNEEZING
- RUNNY NOSE
- ITCHY WATERY EYES
- NASAL CONGESTION
- ASTHMA
- SWELLING OF THE MOUTH, TONGUE OR THROAT
- DIARRHEA (ESPECIALLY IN INFANTS)

NOTE: Persistent sinusitis, irritable bowel syndrome and arthritic-ike pains may also be symptoms of a masked allergy.

Allergies afflict the majority of people in some form or another. Many individuals however, are unaware that certain discomforts nd symptoms can stem from an allergic reaction.

SYMPTOMS NOT NORMALLY ASSOCIATED WITH ALLERGIES

RESPIRATORY SYSTEM: Symptoms may manifest themselves as:

Asthma	Mouth breathing	Shortness of breath
Coughs	Nose bleeds	Tightness in chest
Frequent colds	Post nasal drip	Rattling sounds in
Hayfever	Wheezing	chest
Sinusitis		

Respiratory allergies are often triggered by milk and wheat products and inhalants such as pollens.

CEREBRAL (NERVOUS SYSTEM):

Until recently, the notion that an allergic reaction could affe
the brain was not accepted. There is reason to believe that som
types of allergies can contribute to schizophrenia, depressio
hallucinations, delusions, catatonia, etc. In these cases, th
symptoms are caused by a swelling of the lining of the brair
Clinical ecologists (allergy doctors who take into consideration th
physical, mental, emotional, environmental, etc., reactions t
substances), have been able to help some patients with thes
problems.

Apparently, an array of substances such as auto exhaust, corr
plastic, paint fumes etc., can trigger these symptoms in sensitiv
people. Many so-called mentally ill individuals have been able t
control their symptoms by identifying specific elements whicl
cause their allergic responses and eliminating them. Cerebrall
related allergies are believe to also cause:

Anxiety	Insomnia	Restlessness
Dizzy spells	Learning disorders	Fatigue
Nervousness	Migraines	Crying
Learning problems	Drowsiness	Anger
Memory problems	Anxiety	Lack of concentration
Mental dullness	Irritability	Restlessness
Depression	Hyperactivity	Convulsions

GASTROINTESTINAL SYSTEM:

Some studies have found that 80% of respiratory allergies are
also accompanied by gastrointestinal symptoms. These allergies
can cause the same symptoms as certain gastrointestinal disorder
such as duodenal ulcers, colitis, and appendicitis. Allergies to
certain foods can cause the following symptoms:

Heartburn	Vomiting	Intestinal gas
Indigestion	Diarrhea	Gall Bladder problems
Nausea	Constipation	
Food cravings		

Undigested proteins can act as irritants in the body. T-cells can treat them as foreign invaders, thus inviting an allergic reaction. An efficient digestive (gastro) capability is necessary to prevent accumulations of these substances in the bloodstream.

Mucous membranes line many areas of the body including the nose, throat, most organs and glands, and the gastrointestinal tract. Healthy mucous membranes will not allow undigested proteins to enter the bloodstream.

THE COLON CONNECTION

The colon plays a vital role in maintaining the health of the body. Its function is to eliminate wastes. However, due to faulty eating habits so typical of our society, the colon can become congested or constipated. Consequently, it can harbor all kinds of undischarged toxins, which can poison the body if released into the bloodstream. This state of intestinal toxemia lowers the immune capability of the body and sets the stage for allergies to occur.

NOTE: Allergic symptoms can result from a poorly functioning colon or from contact with certain toxic substances and can cause:

Acne	Dark circles under	Hives
Blisters	the eyes	Itching
Blotches	Eczema	Psoriasis
Flushing		

THE LIVER'S ROLE

The liver can be considered the caretaker of the immune system. It has the critical function of detoxifying the body and can help prevent physiological stressors from causing allergies and disease. Exposure to harmful pollutants, alcohol or malnutrition can weaken the liver and inhibit its function. As a result, toxins are not properly filtered and disposed from the body's cellular system.

CARDIOVASCULAR SYSTEM:

Sometimes, in the case of a food allergy, the cardiovascul, system can be affected. Some people who eat a particular foc which they cannot tolerate can experience the followin symptoms:

Hypertension	High or low blood pressure	Rapid pulse

MUSCULAR/SKELETAL SYSTEM:

Often symptoms which affect the muscles or bones ar triggered by food intolerances. Common offenders include refined sugar and flour, potatoes and tomatoes.

Arthritis	Joint pain	Neck and back ache
Muscle cramps	Muscle fatigue	Shoulder ache
Spasms	Sluggishness	Coordination problems

EARS:

Symptoms of an allergy which affect the ears are also usually linked to a food allergy and can also accompany respiratory symptoms commonly seen with typical allergic reactions.The mos common food allergens associated with ear problems are: wheat, sugar, milk, and chocolate products, as well as pollens and other inhalants.

Frequent ear infections	Imbalance	Loss of hearing
Itching inside ears	Popping of ears	Recurring earaches
Dizziness	Hypersensitivity to noise	

THE ADRENAL GLANDS AND ALLERGIES

The adrenals are two small glands located above the kidneys. Their job is to release hormones which neutralize undigested proteins, and render them harmless. Histamines are released from mast cells whenever the presence of an allergen is detected by the body's immune system. Histamine is the culprit compound which causes inflammation, itching, the flow of mucous etc. The adrenals and liver are responsible for producing natural antihistamines which serve to control this inflammatory response.

DISEASES WHICH HAVE BEEN LINKED TO ALLERGIES

Celiac disease, multiple sclerosis, diabetes, hypoglycemia, epilepsy, bulimia, anorexia, candida and obesity have also been associated with or traced to allergies. Surprisingly enough, addictions are thought to have a link with allergies as well. Stephen Levine, Ph.D., has made this observation: Allergy or allergic-like sensitivities nearly always accompany addiction. An allergy may occur without addiction but, generally, addiction is always accompanied by allergy. Alcoholics, smokers, and avid coffee drinkers are allergic to the very substances they crave. Allergy-Addiction Syndrome is the term used to describe this phenomenon. Addiction-prone individuals, because of their basic physiological makeup, are more likely to overuse cigarettes, coffee, milk, wheat, or common foods to satisfy their constant need for stimulation. Any subtle signal of withdrawal symptoms triggers the individual to eat the necessary food or to light up a cigarette. The increasing addictive nature of these substances continue and create a vicious cycle. When an individual forces himself to give up one substance; alcohol for example, he may in compensation, increase his consumption of coffee, cigarettes, or addictive foods. In this manner, the stimulated state is maintained and withdrawal symptoms avoided. Only when regular consumption of all addictive substances are stopped can a symptom-free state be established. The best testing procedure involves a single-food rotation diet where a particular food is avoided until a full four-day period has elapsed. After four days without the addictive substance, the body can regain its normal ability to discriminate an allergen from an addictant.

CANDIDA: Candiasis refers to a condition in which the yeast organism proliferates and can causes infection in various parts of the body. Candida lives primarily in moist environments including the mouth, throat, intestines and genito-urinary tracts of most humans. When the organism is allowed to reproduce and overgrowth occurs, it can cause a myriad of distressing symptoms. The presence of a yeast infection can cause food and chemical allergies, as well as aggravate existing ones. The main underlying reason for the presence of candiasis is a compromised immune system.

The following play an integral role in combating conditions which lead to allergies.

CHILDREN AND ALLERGIES:

Dr. Marshall Mandell, who wrote the book, *Dr. Mandell's Five Day Allergy Relief System*, became interested in allergic children while working as a pediatrician. He outlines a number of symptoms in children which are attributed to allergies. They include:

Dyslexia	Anger	Mental confusion
Perceptual disorder	Restlessness	Withdrawn attitude
Minimal brain	Headache	Depression
Disorder	Fatigue	Visual blurring
Flushing	Abdominal pain	Lack of concentration
Hyperactivity	Growing pains	Drowsiness
Irritability	Changes in bedwetting	Itching
Penmanship	Changes in speech	Inability to read

BEDWETTING:

Nocturnal Enuresis which persists beyond the age of three is suspected of being caused by allergies. Major allergens which commonly cause problems in children include: (I) milk and milk products; (2) wheat; (3) egg; (4) corn; (5) chocolate; and (6) pork.

Inhalants such as pollens, house dust, molds, and animal hairs have also been implicated in bedwetting. Interestingly, some bedwetters have decreased bladder capacities believed to be caused by an allergic reaction. Allergies cause fluid buildup in the layers of the bladder, which can result in swelling. Theoretically, when the offending food is removed, the child's bladder capacity should return to normal. Recurrent cystitis has been also been linked to food allergy.

HYPERACTIVITY:

Doris I. Rapp, M.D., has extensively studied the association between allergies and hyperactivity in children. Her studies found that children suffering from hyperactivity or Attention Deficit Disorder cannot sit still, have trouble concentrating, cannot control their emotions, don't speak normally, have poor dispositions, may lack affection, sleep poorly and can act aggressively. The consumption of white sugar and certain dyes and food additives are believed to initiate these types of symptoms in some children who are allergic to these substances.

TRADITIONAL MEDICAL AND NON-MEDICAL APPROACHES TO ALLERGY TREATMENT

The medical approach to treating allergies has long been the exclusive domain of traditional allergists. Injection therapy has been the standard mode of treatment since 1911, when it was first introduced. Extracts of an allergen are administered in slowly increasing doses until hopefully, the person develops an immunity to that allergen. This method operates on somewhat the same principle as vaccinations.

Typically, with this type of immunotherapy, shots are given once or twice a week and are gradually reduced to once a month, usually ending after three years. The allergist must use caution when administering these shots, because an accidental overdose could trigger anaphylactic shock, an condition that can be fatal. Because of the risks involved with allergy shots, many allergists rarely give them to children with food allergies. The shots only offer temporary relief for about a third of patients. Another third report permanent relief from symptoms with shot therapy, and the remaining third have recurrences from within a year to 5 to 10 years after treatment. Initially, allergies are detected by a skin test, although this test is not very reliable. Minute injections of extracts of the suspected allergen are placed under the skin of the arms or back. The likely allergen is the one that produces the biggest weal. Frequently, these tests are inconclusive. If the orthodox approach fails to ease the allergy, the only alternatives (at least in the past) have been to use antihistamine or anti-inflammatory drugs, which come with a number of side effects.

Theron G. Randolph, is considered the father of clinical ecology, which is a branch of allergy treatment not strictly confined to antigen-antibody therapy. Antigens (foreign proteins) are the allergy-invoking substances, and antibodies are the entities which attack them, promoting an inflammatory reaction, or allergic response. IgE is the antibody involved in the allergic response.

Allergy victims usually have much more IgE in their blood than most people. Substances exists, (such as environmental chemicals), however, which trigger allergic manifestations which do not cause elevated levels of IgE in the blood. Traditional allergists limit their work only to responses which are mediated by IgE. Clinical ecologists take every possible substance into consideration as allergen suspects. Dr. Randolph states: "The important thing is to diagnose specifically the patient sitting in front of me at the time. I take the history and do what I can to alleviate, arrest, and treat his symptoms effectively. And that is not by means of drugs, which most of the allergists are moving toward, but by means of diagnosing specifically the environmental exposures to which the patient is extremely susceptible and highly reactive."

Many people have been able to find allergy relief even after they have unsuccessfully tried conventional therapies. Apparently, some of us react wildly to specific chemicals in food and the environment, causing all kind of physical and even mental symptoms.

Less traumatic and more reliable than traditional patch tests, the application of sublingual extracts has seen some dramatic results. These extracts, which are readily absorbed into the body, cause an immediate reaction if the person is sensitive to a particular chemical in the extract. Extracts can contain a wide range of chemicals of suspected allergens, from auto exhaust fumes to pineapples. Each extract, however, contains just one specific allergen or chemical in order to pinpoint the offending substance. Traditional allergists oppose this method of diagnosis, claiming that it has no scientific validity. Patients who have finally found answers to their anguish after spending much money exploring other possibilities, tend to disagree emphatically.

TESTING FOR ALLERGIES

The menus and recipes found at the end of this book are suggested as guidelines. If you suspect you are allergic to any of the foods listed, substitute other recipes. If you wish to follow a rotation diet, you would eat a certain food only once every four days. Members of the same food group or family can be used on alternate days. This is a good way to control allergic responses, while you are fortifying your adrenal glands and immune system. Vary your foods as much as possible.

If you're not sure if you are allergic to a certain food, you can give yourself a simple pulse test. This is accomplished by relaxing, then taking your wrist pulse for sixty seconds. Record the number of beats. Eat the suspect food. After 15-20 minutes take your pulse again. If it increases more than ten beats per minute, eliminate that food for one month. Alter one month, test again. A normal pulse reading falls between 52-70 beats. If you desire, you can also record your blood pressure after eating a certain food to test for fluctuations. Kinesiology (muscle-testing) is another easy way to determine food sensitivities.

GOOD HEALTH AND ALLERGIES

It is essential that we keep our immune systems healthy. However when we slip into poor dietary habits or experience significant stress, our natural defenses can malfunction. Normally, when foreign invaders (allergens) are breathed in, the healthy immune system takes care of them via the mucous membranes. The sinuses transport these allergens down the throat where they travel to the digestive tract. This efficient method of removal neutralizes and disposes of foreign substances. The tonsils, adenoids, and lymphatic system each play an important role in the process of eliminating these harmful substances.

Everyone comes in contact with foreign agents on a daily basis Microorganisms such as bacteria, viruses and fungi, environmental chemicals and pollutants, pollen, mold etc continually assault our bodies. An individual can become more vulnerable to these substances when the body is weakened by disease, stress or malnutrition.

Allergies have escalated over the last few decades. Interestingly, the incidence of allergies was significantly lower when nations were agriculturally-based. As industrial technology developed, chemicals, pollutants, food additives, herbicides, pesticides, synthetic drugs, and food stripped of its nutrition appeared. Considering the enormous onslaught of new and potentially damaging compounds we encounter daily, is it any wonder our immune systems have been overly taxed?

COMMON SENSE CARE FOR ALLERGIES

- Avoid foods, plants, animals, drugs, dust or other substances that you know trigger the allergy

- Use a face mask when doing chores

- Get rid of old rugs, pillows, and stuffed animals

- Install an air purifier and air conditioner

- Change the air filter on your furnace frequently

- Don't smoke

- Avoid using aspirin which has been reported to allow food allergens to be more effectively absorbed by the body

- Avoid corn, wheat, eggs, yeast, dairy products, citrus fruits and food additives until you know what the culprit substances are

HERBS FOR ALLERGIES

Nature has provided us with a marvelous assortment of botanicals which help the body cope with allergic reactions. As with any type of medicine, herbs should be used judiciously and ideally with the consent of your doctor.

EPHEDRA/MA HUANG: Ephedra is used for a number of respiratory problems. The natural ephedrine contained in this herb acts as a bronchial-dilator and decongestant.

For this reason, Ephedra is considered a natural antihistamine. The Chinese have used this herb for generations to treat symptoms of asthma and flu. Ephedra must be taken in reasonable doses and not overused.

ALFALFA: Alfalfa helps to assimilate protein, calcium and other nutrients. It is beneficial for all ailments because of nutrient content. Alfalfa is considered a body cleanser and infection fighter. In addition, it provides essential minerals necessary to combat allergies.

ECHINACEA: This herb stimulates the immune system and increases the body's ability to resist infection. It aids in the production of white blood cells and improves lymphatic filtration. Echinacea facilitates the removal of dead cells, toxic bacteria, and foreign material. Echinacea is also rich in iron, zinc, selenium, manganese, silicon and vitamin B-2.

COMFREY: Comfrey helps promote the secretion of pepsin and is a general aid to digestion. It is also excellent healer for respiratory disorders. It is rich in protein, sodium, iron and vitamin A. Comfrey also contains moderate amounts of lysine, which helps control herpes.

GARLIC: Garlic stimulates the lymphatic system to throw off waste matter. It is considered a natural antibiotic. Garlic is rich in selenium, and high in sulphur which acts to protect the immune system.

LICORICE: Licorice works to stimulate the adrenal glands which help to control the histamine which is released during an allergic reaction. Licorice also helps to eliminate excess fluid from the body and helps the body cope with stress. Licorice is high in calcium and potassium. It stimulates hormone production and inhibits tumor growth.

MARSHMALLOW: Marshmallow helps soothe inflamed mucous membranes and expectorate phlegm. It is useful for asthma and other respiratory conditions. Licorice is considered a powerful anti-inflammatory and anti-irritant for the joints and gastrointestinal tract. It is rich in magnesium, iron, selenium and vitamin A.

MULLEIN: Mullein has the ability to loosen mucus and move it out of the body. For this reason, it is recommended for any type of lung or sinus irritation. In addition, Mullein contains antiseptic properties. It is rich in iron, calcium, manganese, potassium, sulphur and niacin.

RED CLOVER: Red Clover acts as a blood purifier and tonic for the nerves. It is useful for coughs, wheezing, bronchitis, and exhaustion. Red Clover contains high amounts of calcium, magnesium, potassium, and vitamin C.

RED RASPBERRY: This plant has a high vitamin and mineral content and is good for anyone who suffers from food allergies. Red Raspberry boosts digestion.

HORSERADISH: Horseradish can help to clear blocked nasal passages and clean the system of infection. It is also considered a natural antihistamine. This herb is rich in sulphur which helps to protect the immune system. Significant amounts of vitamin C and potassium are also found in Horseradish.

ROSE HIPS: Rose Hips are rich in vitamin C, which acts as a natural antihistamine in the body and helps to maintain cell integrity which can be weakened by the presence of allergens. Cells that leak release histamine and aggravate allergic inflammation.

LOBELIA: Lobelia has been traditionally used to relieve bronchial spasms and is preferred for the treatment of bronchitis and congestion. It also acts as a natural expectorant to move mucus out of the body.

GOLDEN SEAL: The root of the Golden Seal plant provides an excellent natural remedy for mucous conditions in the nasal, bronchial, throat, intestines, stomach and bladder areas. It is also a natural antibiotic. NOTE: Golden Seal should be used with caution if you suffer from any type of ragweed allergy.

BURDOCK: Burdock acts as a blood purifier that can facilitate the clearing of toxin through the lymphatic system. Burdock has been used specifically to treat hay fever.

SLIPPERY ELM: Slippery Elm acts as a buffer against irritations and inflammations of the mucous membranes. In addition, it helps to boost the activity of the adrenal glands. It is an excellent remedy for the respiratory system and works to eliminate mucus from the body. Slippery Elm lozenges are good for dry, irritated or sore throats.

BEE POLLEN: Bee Pollen can help to gradually modify allergic reactions to pollens and build immunity. It must be initially taken in very small amounts to determine if a sensitivity exists. If there is none, a slow increase in dosage can occur. Bee pollen contains protein, B- complex vitamins, and vitamins A, D, C and E.

PROTEIN DIGESTIVE AID: The digestive system needs hydrochloric acid to break down protein in the body. Digestive problems can be linked to allergies and seem to occur if digestive enzymes are not doing their job in properly breaking down food. Using a supplement which contains Hydrochloric acid, bromelain or papain is recommended.

HERBAL LOWER BOWEL TONIC: An excellent combination of herbs which will boost colon function and serve to cleanse the bowel consists of the following: Cascara Sagrada, Raspberry Leaves, Lobelia, Turkey Rhubarb,Golden Seal Root, Fennel, and Cayenne (capsicum).

HERBAL LIVER CLEANSE: A combination of herbs which will strengthen the liver are: Alfalfa, Dandelion, Cascara Sagrada, Yellow Dock, Golden Seal Root, Bayberry, Oregon Grape Root, Red Beet Root, Milk Thistle and Lobelia.

NERVE FORMULA: A significant amount of allergies have been linked to nervous disorders. The nervous system can be strengthened by using nervine herbs such as Hops, Scullcap, Valerian, and Passion Flower.

NUTRITIONAL APPROACH TO ALLERGIES

Before any treatment plan for allergies can be incorporated, an inventory of one's dietary habits is essential. Certain foods including: white flour, white sugar, chocolate, dairy products, wheat, potatoes,caffeine, shellfish, citrus fruits and strawberries should be eliminated. In addition, any FD&C yellow #5 dyes, BHT-BHA, monsodium glutamate (MSG) or vanillin should not be consumed.

A diet that is high in whole grains like oats, brown rice and millet, fresh raw stone fruits and vegetables and lean sources of protein like beans and legumes is recommended. Eating at least 25 to 30 grams of fiber is a must to keep the colon well functioning and drinking plenty of pure water is essential. The following vitamins and mineral supplements are also recommended to control allergic reactions.

VITAMIN A: This vitamin helps fortify cells and protects the tissues, especially those found in the respiratory tract. Vitamin A helps to shield cells from the irritation of foreign substances such as pollens. It works best when combined with vitamin E. Vitamins A and E are considered antioxidants which help defend cell membranes from free radical damage. It has been speculated that free radical damage to cells allows allergens to more freely enter the cell structure and cause an allergic reaction.

VITAMIN E: Vitamin E boosts immunity by strengthening cell integrity. It is also a powerful antioxidant and helps to keep tissues oxygenated and healthy.

B-COMPLEX: The B vitamins are essential for the health of the adrenals and the nervous system. Pantothenic acid helps facilitate the production of natural cortisone which is very important in controlling the inflammation of allergies. It is always wise to increase this particular B-vitamin when you are under stress, illness, or suspect the onset of allergies. In addition, B-complex is needed for the production of digestive enzymes in the body.

VITAMIN C: Vitamin C and substances called bioflavonoids act as natural antihistamines and help to detoxify foreign substances entering the body. Vitamin C helps block allergic reactions and rebuilds healthy membranes, especially when combined with the B vitamins and bioflavonoids. Nutrition expert Carlson Wade says, "Also known as ascorbic acid, vitamin C is vital to collagen formation. Collagen is the connective tissue substance that is needed to build immunity to free radicals..."

BIOFLAVONOIDS: These substances, found in the white part of citrus rinds and also in some vitamin C supplements, enhance the availability of vitamin C to the body and aid in its utilization. It also strengthens capillary walls.

CALCIUM: This mineral cleanses the blood, helps regulate the heartbeat, alleviates insomnia, and protects the nervous system.

MAGNESIUM: Magnesium should always be used in conjunction with calcium. Half as much of this mineral as calcium (in milligrams) should be taken. Magnesium supports the nervous system and strengthens the adrenals, which can become stressed during allergic reactions.

POTASSIUM: Potassium helps protect cells from leaking vital fluids. This nutrient feeds the nerves and also strengthens the adrenals. It is important to keep a balanced potassium/sodium ratio in the body. An excess of sodium and a lack of potassium is more commonly seen. Sodium intake should be monitored and if becomes excessive, then supplement your diet with potassium. Herbs rich in potassium include Kelp, Watercress, Horsetail, and Alfalfa.

ZINC: Zinc is an important mineral for the immune system. It strengthens the thymus gland, which is responsible for the production of T-lymphocytes. Zinc is also healing to the mucus membranes.

EVENING PRIMROSE OIL: The fatty acids contained in this oil are needed to produce adrenal hormones. Evening Primrose Oil acts as an over-all stimulant to the immune system.

PREVENTING ALLERGIES

- DO NOT INTRODUCE COW'S MILK, CITRUS JUICES, EGGS, MEATS, NUTS OR WHEAT TOO EARLY INTO AN INFANT'S DIET.

- BREAST FEED INFANTS WHENEVER POSSIBLE FOR AT LEAST SIX MONTHS.

- KEEP YOUR IMMUNE SYSTEM STRONG BY AVOIDING JUNK FOODS, CAFFEINE, TOBACCO, ALCOHOL, WHITE SUGAR, SALT, AND WHITE FLOUR FOODS.

- TAKE A GOOD VITAMIN C WITH BIOFLAVONOID SUPPLEMENT EVERY DAY

- EAT LOTS OF HIGH FIBER FOODS AND DRINK PLENTY OF PURE WATER

CASE HISTORY

I was born as the oldest child in a family of one brother and two sisters. At first, I was the healthiest child in my family. I had very few colds. I remember a lot of aches and pains in my legs that the doctors all called growing pains. I was checked for appendicitis (due to a pain in my right side) so many times the doctor finally showed my dad how to check me.

My mom says I was the healthiest child she had until I turned 13. Then I came down with hay fever in May. By August, it turned into asthma and bronchial pneumonia. This was in 1956. I continued fighting these problems. In August 1959, we moved into a new home. In the process of sweeping cement floors, I began wheezing violently. I was taken to the hospital and received a huge shot. The next three days were spent running to the doctor for more of them. He told my folks that I should be taken to a larger allergy clinic in Salt Lake City.

My first visit was expensive, to say the least. They found I was allergic to my own bacteria and could not have my own allergy tests. This first visit cost my folks over $400.00. That did not include my shot serum, which had to be purchased two to three times a year. To save money, the doctors let my dad give me my shots. I had three shots a week, then two a week, then one a week.

My husband and I were married in 1963, and he was taught how to give me my shots. I lived a fairly normal life until we tried having a family. I was having urinary problems and the doctor learned I was allergic to chlorine. He put dye through a tube directly into my kidneys. He found I had acute cystitis. I took sulfa pills for awhile to help it and then the urologist tried another method with silver nitrate. They gave me a shot through my urethra right into the wall of my bladder. I would rather have a baby than undergo the pain of silver nitrate treatment. I was pregnant. However, two days after the test, I miscarried.

It took me until December of 1965 to finally get pregnant again. The baby was due in August of 1966. I felt great all through my pregnancy, until July. I was taking water pills for fluid retention, but one morning I woke up with my face swollen. The doctor checked me and sent me straight to the hospital. I had toxemia and my blood pressure was so high that they gave me a pill in the morning and I slept until two that afternoon. I was so drugged I made no sense. My brain would attempt to stimulate an action, but my body would not respond. I was so nauseated I couldn't eat. I lived on baked potatoes and lettuce the last month of my pregnancy. The baby had a good strong heartbeat, but eventually the doctors failed to find it. They sent me to the hospital for x-rays and found that the baby was dead. Three weeks later, in September of 1966, we adopted our first baby, David. He was born out-of-state and some people thought he was the baby I had been pregnant with. Six months later, I became pregnant again, but we lost this one too.

About the time the baby would have been born we adopted Sara. She was born with a full-cleft palate, and we loved her like she was our natural child. Believe it or not, our two adopted kids were both born with hay fever and asthma. When David was three months old (in December 1966), the doctors put him in the hospital and forced him onto soy meat and milk. From then until he outgrew his asthma at puberty, his allergies always affected his stomach and intestines. By the time he was 2-1/2 years old, he had diarrhea so bad he bled. By the time David was three years old, he was on one gamma shot and three allergy shots a week.

The Lord blessed me through these years with good health to take care of my kids and their problems. In fact, my health improved so much I got pregnant without even trying. This was a surprise pregnancy, and so I decided I would make every effort I could to see that this baby made it. I had felt for some time that my husband and I were meant to adopt our children instead of having our own. I decided whatever happened with this pregnancy would be my answer from the Lord. If I had the baby we could try having more of our own, and if not, we were to adopt all of our children. Six weeks from my due date I experienced heavy hemorrhaging. I was taken to the hospital and had an emergency D&C. The baby died a few hours later.

In 1971, we filed papers with immigration to get a daughter from Korea. I experienced an asthma attack. My family doctor did not accept the fact that my asthma was a result of an allergic reaction. To him it was more stress-related, and if I tried hard enough, I could control it. He gave me a cortisone shot and I was on top of the world that whole day. But by the next day, I was so depressed all I could do was cry. I could not snap out of it. I even felt suicidal. The doctor heard what my reactions were and did not want anything to do with me. He sent me to my asthma doctor. He was out-of-town so David's pediatric allergist took care of me. He said if I was having reactions to the cortisone all he could do for me was put me in the hospital and give me the drug through an IV drip.

In August of 1971, I made my third trip to the hospital in six months. I was a nervous wreck. I wanted to go home and told the doctor I would get well faster there than in the hospital. Our daughter arrived from Korea in December of 1971. She was nine months old. This is when my health really took a turn for the worse. David and Sara had to help me with Loni when my husband wasn't home because of my lack of energy. In the spring of 1972, when hay fever season hit, I started on my sinus medication and then started having more bladder problems. When I went to the urologist, I could not empty anything out of my bladder. The nurse catherized me and drained over a quart out of my bladder. She advised me not take the medication anymore.

In October of 1973 Robert came to us from Korea. He was 4-1/2 years old. He had been abandoned in Korea one month before he had turned four. Robert weighed 22 pounds. By the spring of 1974, we discovered we had adopted four children, all of whom had some form of hay fever and asthma. So, not only did we have to deal with my health problems, but four others as well.

At this time, four out of the six of us were on allergy shots. An allergy clinic opened up locally, so I made one last trip to the allergy clinic in Salt Lake City. I remember it well. They gave me 36 shots, just under the skin up each side of my arms. When the doctor saw my arm, he told her to get the cortisone cream. They brought me an allergy pill with antihistamine in it to take care of the swelling and itching.

In fall of 1977, I had another asthma attack and had to go into the hospital again for another cortisone treatment. It only took a few days and I was over the attack, however I had to face terrible cortisone withdrawal again.

In 1979 I started having chest pains and being short of breath. I was placed on Valium and two different kinds of antidepressants and sent on my way. By now, I was on three antihistamine-type hay fever pills, three asthma pills, three Valium and six of two different kinds of antidepressants, a total of fifteen hard chemical drugs a day. I developed an esophageal ulcer and a hiatal hernia and wound up in the hospital again and experienced another asthma attack.

I was in and out of hospitals constantly. At one point, my bladder shut down and I had to wear a catheter. I had to wear it for five days. When I took the catheter out, I vowed I would never go through that again. I had to be on bladder pain pills just to be able to stand it. I knew there were other ways, and I just had to find them. I knew the best doctor I could find was the Lord. I decided to pray for new direction. That was the best decision I have ever made, and that was a big turning point in my life.

I was directed to a health practitioner, who introduced me to massage therapy for the lymph system, colonics and herbs. I felt so much better through this treatment that I was able to eat good foods I hadn't been able to eat for years.

Another practitioner was even able to pull the old cortisone out of my system, as well as all the other drugs I had been given. Through him, I found out I not only had pollen allergies and food allergies, but chemical and industrial allergies as well. I am allergic to formaldehyde and it is found in everything from carpets to wall paneling, to paint and furniture. I saw this practitioner for two years. He discovered I had Candida. We found we could trace almost all my problems right back to a yeast infection. This was in the spring of 1984, and I have been on various stages of the strict Candida diet and the lesser diet ever since. I am using a Candida nutritional supplement with acidophilus and Pau d'arco.

The problem I am having now is caused by air pollution which results in such bad asthma attacks that some days I must take asthma medication. When I do, I look pregnant by the end of the day. Even with the problems I am still having, I feel better than when I was on chemical drugs. You can endure anything when you can see a light at the end of the tunnel.

I am hoping that when I get the Candida completely under control, more of my problems will ease up. I know that it will still take time.

MENUS AND RECIPES

Some of the following recipes are taken from *Today's Healthy Eating* by Louise Tenney and are designated by asterisks. These recipes are part of an elimination diet which can help to identify certain foods that may be causing allergic reactions.

Diet to Check for Milk Allergy

#1 Breakfast

Oatmeal with Nut Milk*
Sliced Banana

#1 Lunch

` Rye Bread* with Tuna
Alfalfa Sprouts
Mock Mayonnaise*
Carrot Sticks

#1 Supper

Chili
Sesame Bread Sticks*
Garden Salad*

Diet to Check for Wheat Allergy

#2 Breakfast

Raw Granola #1*
NutMilk*
Pure Grape Juice

#2 Lunch

Vegetable Stir Fry*
Beverage

#2 Supper

Steamed Chicken Breast
Steamed Broccoli
10 Almonds, raw

Diet to Check for Sugar Allergy

#3 Breakfast

Poached Egg
Toast
Juice, unsweetened

#3 Lunch

Lentil and Nut Dish
Fresh Carrot Juice
Lettuce/Sprouts/Green Onion
Salad w/lemon juice

#3 Supper

Cheese Enchiladas*
Fresh Avocado Salad*

Diet to Check for Egg Allergy

#4 Breakfast

Yogurt and Fruit*

#4 Lunch

Vegetable Broth #2*
Rye Bread*

#4 Supper

BeanLo*
Brown Rice
Beverage

Diet to Check for Corn Allergy

#5 Breakfast

Cottage Cheese with 2 fruits of
choice Whole Grain Toast
w/pure butter

#5 Lunch

Cooked Lean Beef Patty
w/sauteed onion slices
Steamed Carrot Slices
Brown Rice

#5 Supper

Alfalfa/Artichoke Salad*
Bran Muffins*
Citrus-Free Diet

#6 Breakfast

Blueberry Muffins*
Poached Egg
Apple/Chamomile Drink*

#6 Lunch

Dried Pea Soup*
Sesame Bread Sticks*

#6 Supper

Pecan Celery Patties*
Baked Potato
Beverage

#7 Breakfast

Raw Oat Cereal*
Beverage

#7 Lunch

Brussels Sprouts Casserole*
Brown Rice

#7 Supper

Baked Fish (your choice)
Parsley Garnish
Pineapple Waldorf Salad*

RECIPES

ALMOND (Nut) MILK

1 C. almonds, ground 1 qt. pure water
2 T. pure maple syrup

Blend thoroughly in a blender until smooth. Strain through a strainer or cheese cloth.

RYE BREAD

4 T. dry yeast
1 1/2 C. molasses
6 C. warm water
1 C. wheat germ
2 T. sea salt or salt substitute

5 C. rye flour
10 C. whole wheat flour
4 T. lecithin
8 T. cold pressed oil

Dissolve 4 T. dry yeast into a mixture of 1 1/2 C. molasses and 6 C. warm water. Add 2 T. sea salt, 5 C. rye flour and 3 C. whole wheat flour. Blend well. Beat at least 100 times (very important)! Let stand for about 20 minutes. Mix in 8 T. cold-pressed oil and gradually blend in the remaining 7 C. (about) of whole wheat flour. Knead, cover, and let rise for about 1/2 hour. Should double in bulk. Do not let dough rise too high. Form into 4 large loaves, place in greased loaf pans and let rise for about 1/2 hour. Bake in 350F. oven for about 1 hour.

CASHEW MAYONNAISE

1 1/2 C. raw cashews
1 C. pure water
1 tsp. kelp or mineral salt
4 T. fresh lemon juice
1 T. lecithin

1/2 tsp. paprika
1/4 tsp. powdered mustard
1 C. safflower oil

Blend the first 6 ingredients. Add lemon slowly. Pour the oil, while blender is running, in a thin stream. Chill.

RAW GRANOLA #1

6 C. raw oatmeal (baby oats)	1 C. shredded coconut
1 C. ground sunflower seeds	1 C. ground almonds
1 C. ground sesame seeds	1-1/2 tsp. grated orange rind
1/4 C. ground chia seeds	1/2 tsp. cardamom
1 C. flaxseeds, ground	1 C. date sugar
	1/2 C. warm honey

Mix all ingredients together and drip warm honey and stir. The best method is cooking in the oven at 200 F. for about an hour, stirring often. Granola can be kept in a cool dry place or frozen. It acts as an intestinal broom and cleanser.

VEGETABLE STIR FRY

1 C. carrots, sliced	1/2 C. blanched almonds, chopped
1 C. red onions	1/4 C. sunflower seeds
1 C. broccoli, sliced	2 Tbs. soy sauce (natural)
1 C. cauliflower	1/2 tsp. basil
2 cloves garlic, minced	1/4 tsp. cumin

Heat two Tbs. ghee, butter or cold-pressed oil in wok or frying pan. Add carrots, onions, garlic and herbs, stir thoroughly, cover and let cook for five minutes. Stir occasionally and you may add a few tablespoons of water if the vegetables get too dry. Add broccoli and blanched almonds, stir; cover and cook for about 3 minutes. Add cauliflower, sunflower seeds and soy sauce and stir thoroughly. Cover and cook for about ten minutes.

Serve over millet, brown rice or other grain and use vegetables in season such as zucchini, green peppers, Brussels sprouts and cabbage. Add fresh corn, mushrooms or bean sprouts.

CHEESE ENCHILADAS

12 corn tortillas	1 small can tomato sauce
2 C. mild cheese, grated	1 pint sour cream or mock sour cream
1/2 C. onions	
1 small can diced green chilies	Black olives (optional)
1 large can enchilada sauce	

Heat enchilada sauce and tomato sauce with 1 small can of water. Mix the cheese, onions and chilies. Dip tortilla in the hot sauce to soften. Place about 2 T. of the cheese mixture on tortilla, top with a heaping tablespoon of sour cream; roll the tortilla and place seam side down in a baking dish. When all tortillas are rolled up, pour the rest of the enchilada sauce on the top and sprinkle top with cheese and olives. Bake in 350F. oven for about 30 minutes.

SESAME BREAD STICKS (Unleavened)

2 C. sifted whole wheat
   flour
1 T. date sugar or honey
1/2 tsp. sea salt (or omit)

3 T. cold-pressed oil
1/2 tsp. cinnamon
3 1/4 C. cold water

Add all ingredients together and stir well. Knead into little balls. Roll into pencil-like strips 8 inches long and 1/2 inch around. Place on a greased cookie sheet and bake for 30 minutes at 350F.

GARDEN SALAD

3 C. leaf lettuce
1/2 C. fresh peas, shelled
1/2 C. carrots, grated
1/2 C. zucchini, grated

1 C. mung bean sprouts
1 cucumber, sliced
1/2 avocado
1/2 C. mixed sunflower
   seeds and ground almonds

Mix all ingredients together. Serve with herb dressing or dressing of your choice.

FRESH AVOCADO SALAD

2 C. fresh corn, off cob
1 large avocado, diced
2 small tomatoes, diced
1/2 C. green pepper,
   diced

1 T. olive oil
1 tsp. cider vinegar
Kelp and broth seasoning
   to taste

Blend all ingredients together and serve on a bed of leaf lettuce. Top with homemade mayonnaise or salsa.

YOGURT AND FRUIT

2 C. yogurt
2 C. frozen or fresh
1/2 C. ground almonds
blueberries or
strawberries

1 apple, grated
Pure maple syrup

2 ripe bananas, sliced

Fold fruit into yogurt and sweeten with maple syrup to taste. Garnish with ground almonds.

VEGETABLE BROTH #2

6 medium potatoes
4 medium onions
2 ripe tomatoes
2 stalks celery

3 carrots
1 clove garlic
Kelp, vegetable broth
    seasoning to taste
3 qts. pure water

Put all the ingredients in the water, bring to a boil and simmer covered for about one hour. Add herbs of your choice after 45 minutes. Add fresh parsley, basil or thyme. You may want to adjust the quantities of ingredients according to the number of servings you desire.

ALFALFA AND ARTICHOKE SALAD

2 C. alfalfa sprouts
1 C. Jerusalem artichokes
    sliced
1 C. tomatoes, sliced
    lengthwise

1 small avocado, diced
1 small green pepper, diced
1 C. carrots, grated
1 C. celery, chopped

Combine all ingredients together. Good with Italian dressing or one of your choice.

BLUEBERRY MUFFINS

1-3/4 C. whole wheat
    pastry flour
1/4 C. wheat germ
4 tsp. baking powder
    (aluminum free)
1/2 tsp. pure vanilla
1 tsp. sea salt

1 egg
6 T. cold-pressed oil
1/4 C. honey
1 T. lecithin
1 C. sesame milk
1 C. blueberries (fresh
    or frozen

Blend all dry ingredients together. Beat egg, oil, honey and lecithin together and stir into dry ingredients. Add milk and fold in blueberries. Put in greased muffin tins. Bake for about 25 minutes at 375F.

APPLE/CHAMOMILE DRINK

A drink to soothe and calm the nerves.

4 C. raw apple juice
4 C.chamomile tea
1/4 tsp. cinnamon

1/4 tsp. cardamom
1/4 tsp. ginger
Malt sugar to taste

Can be served hot or cold. Enjoy.

DRIED PEA SOUP

1 C. dried split peas
4 C. pure water, cold
1 medium onion, minced
1 C. celery, chopped

2 small carrots, grated
2 T. chopped parsley
1/2 C. nut cream
1 tsp. vegetable salt or
    kelp

Cook the peas in water after soaking overnight. Cook with vegetables for about two hours. When done, add nut cream and seasoning.

PECAN CELERY PATTIES

1 C. pecans
6 stalks celery
3 T. ripe olives
3 green onions

1/4 C. watercress
1/4 C. parsley
1 avocado
Dash of sage or kelp (more
    if needed)

Grind celery, onions, parsley and watercress. Drain the juice.
Grind the pecans fine, mash the avocado, and chop the olives; combine all together and shape into patties. Serve on red leaf lettuce and top with paprika and 1 whole olive.

RAW OAT CEREAL

Eat this cereal for healthy bowel activity.

1 1/2 C. raw oats
1 T. ground almonds
1 T. ground sesame seeds

1 tsp. date sugar
1 T. raisins, soaked in
water

Add bananas, fresh peaches, fresh berries, ground sunflower seeds, sesame seeds, or cashews. Rice polishings, wheat germ, bran etc. can also be added.

BRUSSELS SPROUTS CASSEROLE

1 C. Brussels sprouts
    steamed
1 C. red cabbage, chopped
2 red onions, chopped
2 C. carrots, sliced and
    steamed

1 C. potatoes, skins on,
    diced and steamed
2 T mineral bouillon
1 tsp. mineral salt
1 tsp. kelp
2 T. olive oil
1 C. tomato juice

Combine Brussels sprouts, carrots and potatoes. Add all other ingredients and cover with tomato juice. Cook in oven for 30 minutes at 350 F.

PINEAPPLE WALDORF SALAD

1 C. celery hearts
1 C. apples
1 C. fresh pineapple
Leaf lettuce
1/4 C. chopped walnuts

Raisins (optional)
Homemade mayonnaise

Combine celery hearts, apples, pineapple, nuts and raisins. Add mayonnaise. This salad is also delicious without mayonnaise. Serve on leaf lettuce.

LENTIL AND NUT LOAF

2 C. cooked lentils
1 C. cooked millet
2 medium onions, chopped
1 C. fresh tomatoes,
   blended
1/2 C. almonds, ground

1 tsp. garlic, minced
1 egg
1/2 C. almond milk
1 tsp. kelp or mineral salt

Saute onion in olive oil. Blend lentils, add onions and tomatoes. Mix all other ingredients and pour into oiled loaf pan. Sprinkle parmesan cheese on top. Bake at 350F. for 30 minutes.